INTERMI

FASTING

The complete guide to Intermittent Fasting and the Key to your healthy Weight Loss

BY Melissa White

EDITION 2

UPDATE CHAPTER 4

4

Chapter 1. Current Evidence of Intermittent Fasting in Clinical Practice

Intermittent fasting (IF), or time-confined taking care of, is an arising dietary intercession that limits admission of food and energy for a given period. Not exclusively does this technique confine absolute caloric admission, it likewise advances metabolic homeostasis by supporting circadian taking care of rhythms. Just in the latest 200 years have people had the option to get to provisions of tremendous measures of food and assets, which has caused a change in illness designs, especially for metabolic conditions and corpulence. The possibility that diminishing caloric admission can bring about developmental cell reactions for endurance has been a functioning exploration topic, however with the new open mindfulness and interest in IF, numerous clinical investigations have been distributed all the more as of late. On December 2019, scientists distributed an audit article that talks about the instruments and current clinical proof for IF. This survey article examines different wide range advantages of IF, with an inspirational perspective for more clinical proof later on.

INTERMITTENT FASTING IN CLINICAL PRACTICE

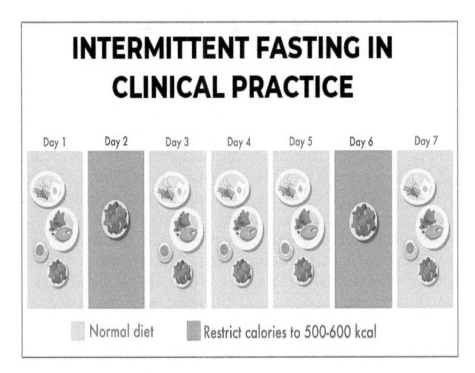

Day 1   Day 2   Day 3   Day 4   Day 5   Day 6   Day 7

Normal diet   Restrict calories to 500-600 kcal

The transition of fuel source from glucose to fatty substances, also known as the "ketogenic diet," is the most widely accepted theory behind the critical physiologic reaction after IF. This metabolic switch increases mitochondrial stress resistance, subterranean insect oxidative defenses, and autophagy while decreasing blood insulin levels. Scientists delineated in their survey that invigorating autophagy while repressing the mammalian objective of rapamycin protein combination pathway can prompt evacuation of oxidative harmed cells. In a survey by scientists IF was appeared to effect memory procurement and intellectual conduct in subject. One potential theory for this impact is creation of master incendiary elements with glucose-based weight control plans. The decrease of these genius fiery variables might be helpful for diminishing foundational irritation and oxidative pressure factors that assume a part being developed of atherosclerosis.

1.1 Introduction

A few clinical examinations, including some randomized control preliminaries, have been performed to break down the impacts of intermittent fasting IF and caloric limitation in a wide scope of uses. Albeit preclinical investigations have exhibited decrease of insulin affectability after caloric limitation and intermittent fasting, clinical examinations have showed conflicting outcomes. The calorie limitation and cardio metabolic danger (CALERIE) study is a stage 2, multicenter, randomized control preliminary where 218 patients were dispensed to either the 25% caloric confining gathering (143) or a not indispensable benchmark group (75). In the confining gathering, there was critical misfortune in body weight and decrease in other cardio metabolic factors like low-thickness lipoprotein (LDL) cholesterol and circulatory strain. Fasting glucose was altogether decreased at the main year, however there was no huge decrease at the subsequent year. Nonetheless, there was a critical diminishing in a substitute marker for insulin obstruction, which was assessed by the homeostatic model appraisal for insulin opposition (HOMA). Another investigation by analysts assessed the recurrence and circadian planning of taking care of with metabolic condition and bosom disease hazard in ladies and showed no relationship of HOMA with evening calorie consumption, eating recurrence, or evening fasting term. As of late, an analyst distributed a solitary arm investigation of 19 patients with metabolic condition who were for the most part on statin as well as antihypertensive treatment. Patients were limited to a 10-hour time of taking care of and were analyzed for body creation and other wellbeing measurements following 12 weeks. There was critical lessening in body weight, muscle versus fat, systolic/diastolic circulatory strain, all out cholesterol, and LDL-cholesterol. In spite of the fact that there was a pattern toward decline of blood glucose and glycosylated hemoglobin (HbA1c) levels, there was no measurably critical advantage. In any case, in a subgroup examination of patients with either raised fasting glucose 100 mg/dL or potentially HbA1c is equivalent to 5.7%, there was a critical decrease in HbA1c level.

Intermittent Fasting IF goes about as a pressure signal trigger, preconditioning cells before ischemic tissue injury. Analysts contrasted subject and a 3-day water-just fasting, multi week without protein fasting, and over nourishment (high-fat eating regimen) diet convention preceding vascular medical procedure. Present moment, 3-day fasting before vascular medical procedure fundamentally constricted intimal hyperplasia and decreased ischemia-reperfusion results. A randomized control preliminary inspected bariatric patients who were planned to go through gastric detour a medical procedure and thought about a 14-day low-calorie diet (VLCD) bunch with the not obligatory benchmark group. Despite the fact that there was no distinction in activity time, the quantity of 30-day difficulties was higher in the benchmark group than the VLCD bunch. Stomach a medical procedure expansions in trouble with expanding muscle versus fat organization, and high measures of instinctive fat lead to messy analyzing of the body planes, bringing about a usable field inclined to irritation and liquid assortment. Moreover, high subcutaneous fat convolutes wound conclusion, bringing about more continuous injury intricacies.

The potential advantages of intermittent fasting IF before elective medical procedure are right now dubious, particularly contrasted and the Enhanced Recovery after Surgery (ERAS) convention, which is currently being executed with acceptable results in different sorts of a medical procedure. One of the well-known segments of the ERAS program is diminishing preoperative fasting time to 6 hours and giving oral carb answers for as long as 2 hours before medical procedure empowering preoperative oral sustenance. This hypothetically diminishes preoperative uneasiness, and patients' progress into an anabolic state to profit by postoperative sustenance. The ERAS convention is a complete thought for decreasing careful pressure to advance quicker recuperation; notwithstanding, it doesn't investigate fasting alone. In this way, the current accomplishment of the ERAS conventions may not really be owing to diminished preoperative fasting, and extra all around planned control contemplates are expected to explain what preoperative fasting means for patient result.

Notwithstanding all the arising proof, there are still a few entanglements and useful troubles to intermittent fasting IF and caloric limitation that are consistently being contemplated. To begin with, physiologic examinations have not yet accomplished agreement on the ideal planning for IF. A few examinations have utilized elective day fasting, and some have utilized a day by day time limited timetable. In spite of the fact that reviews have shown that IF decreases patient stress4 in the long haul, most patients think that it's distressing and are hesitant to begin confining admission, diminishing patient consistence. Around the world, particularly in Korea, numerous individuals accept that skirting one of the three suppers in a day will bring about weakening of wellbeing and wholesome equilibrium. To address such basic concerns, analysts recommended that doctors give satisfactory data and persistent help to pertinent patients.

In this period where food is plentiful, researchers must reexamine the thought that "more is better" with regards to sustenance. Notwithstanding the sum investigation in regards to IF in clinical practice, there are numerous zones that have not yet been investigated in all around planned clinical preliminaries. Along these lines, extra examination and thought are expected to streamline patient results.

1.2 The Science of Going without Intermittent Fasting

Many eating regimen and exercise patterns have beginnings in real science, however the realities will in general get contorted when they accomplish standard prominence. Advantages are misrepresented. Dangers are made light of. Science takes a rearward sitting arrangement to showcasing.

One needn't look any farther than the arising pattern of intermittent fasting for a perfect representation. Supporters for taking occasional splits from gobbling for as long as 24 hours a few times per week promote it as a powerful and exploration upheld methods for shedding pounds and improving wellbeing. That message has been arriving at an ever increasing number of ears of late. "At the present time, we are at a truly significant point for fasting," says a specialist on intermittent fasting and writer of the book Eat Stop Eat. "It's getting very mainstream."

So mainstream, truth be told, that it is rapidly moving into trend and area, recommends master. Also, when something turns into a prevailing fashion seriously well known yet just for a brief period a few issues commonly follow. For one, he says, numerous specialists and nourishment specialists are inclined to excusing trends insane. So their patients and customers, while safeguarded from the strange cases of overeager eating fewer carbs evangelists, may likewise miss out on the authentic advantages of fasting done right. You know, the child and bathwater thing.

Another worry is that advertisers of intermittent fasting will, maybe accidentally, empower outrageous conduct, for example, gorging. This is reflected in the photographs going with numerous new articles on "the quick eating routine" or the "5:2 eating regimen." Often, they portray individuals eating piles of unhealthy, high-fat food varieties, like cheeseburgers, French fries and cake. The ramifications being that on the off chance that you quick two days every week, you can eat up however much garbage that your neck can swallow during the excess five days.

There is a huge assemblage of proof that recommends fasting can profit both the body and mind, yet most exploration has been directed on creatures, like subject. Scientists reading fasting are calling for more human investigations.

Not really, say more moderate defenders of fasting. Their interpretation of intermittent fasting: eat reasonably more often than not, eat nothing for an all-inclusive period occasionally, enjoy just every so often (maybe once per week, say, on an assigned "cheat day"). There is research, they guarantee, to back up the medical advantages of reasonably fusing fasting into your way of life.

There is without a doubt a huge collection of examination to help the medical advantages of fasting, however its majority has been led on creatures, not people. All things considered, the outcomes have been promising. Fasting has been appeared to improve biomarkers of illness, diminish oxidative pressure and save learning and memory working, as per senior specialist for the national institute on aging, part of the US national institutes of health. Experts has researched the medical advantages of intermittent fasting on the cardiovascular framework and mind in rodents, and has called for "very much controlled human investigations" in individuals "across a scope of weight lists".

There are a few hypotheses regarding why fasting gives physiological advantages, says master. "The one on which we've focused a lot of attention and planned investigations to test is the theory that cells are under gentle pressure during the fasting period," Expert says.

Despite the fact that "stress" is regularly utilized from a negative perspective, burdening the body and brain has benefits. Think about incredible exercise, which stresses, specifically, muscles and the cardiovascular framework. However long you give your body time to recuperate, it will develop further. "There is significant closeness between how cells react to the pressure of activity and how cells react to intermittent fasting," says specialists.

Specialist has added to a few different examinations on intermittent fasting and caloric limitation. In one, overweight grown-ups with moderate asthma burned-through just 20% of their typical calorie consumption on substitute days. Members who clung to the eating regimen lost 8% of their underlying body weight more than about two months. They likewise saw an abatement in markers of oxidative pressure and aggravation, and improvement of asthma-related manifestations and a few personal satisfaction pointers.

In another examination, analysts investigated the impacts of intermittent and nonstop energy limitation on weight reduction and different biomarkers (for conditions including bosom malignant growth, diabetes and cardiovascular illness) among youthful overweight lady. They tracked down that intermittent limitation was pretty much as successful as persistent limitation for improving weight reduction, insulin affectability and other wellbeing biomarkers.

Master has likewise explored the defensive advantages of fasting to neurons. In the event that you don't eat for 10–16 hours, your body will go to its fat stores for energy, and unsaturated fats called ketones will be delivered into the circulatory system. This has been appeared to ensure memory and learning usefulness, says master, just as sluggish sickness measures in the cerebrum.

However, maybe it isn't such an excess of the fasting that produces medical advantages, essentially, as the subsequent by and large decrease in calorie admission (if, that is, you don't gorge on non-fasting days, which could make a caloric excess rather than a deficiency). That shows up, in any event, to be the situation in easing back infections like malignant growth in subject, as indicated by specialist.

"Caloric limitation, under nourishment without ailing health, is the lone trial approach reliably appeared to draw out endurance in creature models," Researchers expressed in an investigation on the impacts of intermittent fasting on prostate malignancy development in subject. In the examination, subject abstained double seven days for 24 hours, yet were generally allowed to eat at freedom. During non-fasting days, the subject gorged. Generally, they didn't get in shape, checking whatever benefits they may have seen from fasting. Intermittent fasting with compensatory indulging "didn't improve mouse endurance nor did it defer prostrate tumor development," the examination closed.

To improve wellbeing, the objective ought to be to get more fit by lessening the aggregate sum of calories devoured, proposes master, as opposed to zeroing in on when those calories are burned-through. "On the off chance that you [don't] eat two days per week, and cutoff what you eat the other five days, you will get fit. It's one way to deal with getting in shape.

Individuals ought to likewise be careful about books composed for wide crowds that clarify the science behind fasting or some other wellbeing pattern, he says. One reason for composing a book for the buyer market, all things considered, is to sell however many duplicates as could be expected under the circumstances. Creators will in general present just proof supporting their perspective, proposes master, while disregarding proof that negates it.

Chapter 2. The Choice for a Healthier Lifestyle with Intermittent Fasting

Corpulence is an overall pestilence because of the accessibility of numerous unfortunate food alternatives and restricted actual exercise. Limitation of the everyday food consumption brings about weight reduction, which is additionally connected with better wellbeing results including fatty substances, absolute cholesterol, low-thickness lipoprotein cholesterol, circulatory strain, glucose, insulin, and C-receptive protein. Our point is to momentarily examine the impacts of intermittent fasting on weight and other biochemical markers referenced already. The examination is planned as a deliberate audit as indicated by the Preferred Reporting Items for Systematic Reviews and Meta-Analyses agenda. To survey the viability of intermittent fasting, related examinations were explored somewhere in the range of 2000 and 2018 and 815 investigations were recognized. Just four articles met the preset incorporation and avoidance models. Every one of the four examinations have shown a huge reduction in fat mass with P-values 0.01. It was additionally noticed that some biochemical markers were altogether decreased, for example, the decrease in low-thickness lipoprotein and fatty substance with P-values 0.05. Other biochemical markers had conflicting outcomes. In view of the subjective examination, intermittent fasting was discovered to be productive in decreasing weight, regardless of the weight list. Further examinations are expected to survey the capacity to keep up the shed pounds without recapturing it and the drawn out impacts of such dietary changes.

2.1 Background and Introduction

As of late, individuals worldwide have built up an expanded notoriety for health improvement plan, diet plans and weight upkeep programs with little examination done on the adequacy of those projects. In the interim, weight has been expanding in commonness because of numerous social determinants like simple admittance to different quick food sources, and absence of active work. In 2016, World Health Organization (WHO) revealed that more than 1.9 billion individuals on the planet were overweight and more than 650 million individuals were hefty which has significantly increased in number since 1975. Additionally, stoutness is a realized danger factor for some, metabolic problems like coronary illness, malignancies, osteoarthritis and respiratory issues.

INTERMITTENT FASTING
& HEALTHIER LIFESTYLE

According to the meta-investigation done by scientists, it was recommended that way of life changes are quite possibly the best techniques in diminishing weight and the dangers for cardiovascular sicknesses. Weight reduction generally prompts the improvement in the general prosperity of patients and their biomarkers, for example, systolic and diastolic circulatory strain, glucose, insulin, absolute serum cholesterol, fiery biomarkers and low-thickness lipoprotein (LDL). There are numerous types of diet and activities programs accessible for weight reduction, in any case, one of the most un-perceived eating routine changes is the other day fasting (ADF) which incorporates eating 20% of energy prerequisites on a quick day and afterward burn-through food not indispensable on the feed days which has been interesting to be exceptionally powerful for weight reduction.

The point of our precise audit is to sum up the impacts of ADF/intermittent fasting on weight reduction, the effect on biomarkers, and cardiovascular danger factors subsequently surveying it.

2.2 Methods and Review

The plan of the investigation is a quick subjective methodical survey in accordance with the Preferred Reporting Items for Systematic Reviews and Meta-Analyses agenda. A writing audit was performed freely by two commentators. The creators pick a wide scope of web crawlers to utilize. The inquiry was restricted by utilizing the accompanying channels: Human subjects, English language, and since the year 2000. Unimportant distributions were dispensed with from the title of those examinations which did exclude the word fasting or dietary limitation. The current examination depends on a subjective way to deal with evaluating the adequacy of intermittent fasting in diminishing body weight and embracing a better way of life. Consequently, the examination configuration did exclude the estimation of the quantitative measures.

Selection of Study

The incorporation standards for distributions incorporated any distributed article evaluating intermittent fasting in 18-year-old patients or more seasoned, randomized controlled preliminaries, contemplates estimating the impact of intermittent fasting on body weight as an essential result, and weight file. We additionally allocated the Grading of Recommendations Assessment, Development and Evaluation score of four or higher as an assessment proportion of the distributions generally speaking quality. Prohibition models incorporated any examination with members more youthful than 18 years old, any investigation that is definitely not a randomized clinical, and those examinations that didn't score four or higher on the evaluation system. It shows the four chose concentrates with meanings of the intercessions.

Results

The result of interest is the adequacy of intermittent fasting on weight reduction and other biomarkers, while likewise surveying for the general nature of the chose clinical preliminaries to guarantee high subjective orderly audit.

Characteristics Study

The two specialists, aggregately recognized 815 investigations since 2000, which implies a decent strength of arrangement. Of those, 258 articles were taken out since they were copies. Further, 439 investigations were avoided (theoretical, concentrate in progress, orderly surveys, and meta-examination). At that point we evaluated 118 articles for qualification. It shows the PRISMA stream graph. At last, we remembered four randomized controlled preliminaries for our subjective methodical audit. It gives the segment data about the chose considers.

2.3 Outcomes

A randomized controlled preliminary assessed the job of ADF to get in shape in overweight and typical weight people. Subjects had a feed day exchanged with a quick day with 25% of absolute energy admission. Substitute day fasting bunch has an abatement in fat mass by 3.6 kg, C-responsive protein, leptin and triacylglycerol (TG) focuses, expansion in low thickness lipoprotein (LDL) molecule size and plasma adiponectin while leptin diminished when contrasted with the benchmark group. In any case, there was no adjustment of low-thickness lipoprotein, high-thickness lipoprotein, and homocysteine toward the finish of study period. Cases and controls didn't have any issues in clinging to the investigation diet for 12 weeks. Announced hyperphagia on the feed day thusly prompts by and large higher energy limitation all through the investigation period which was a significant reason for the weight reduction. Dietary fulfillment and feeling of feeling completion expanded toward the finish of 12 weeks which may have assumed a part in adherence to abstain from food in the long haul. Not many limits of this investigation were the low number of study subjects (15 patients in each gathering), no active work estimation, and the chance of under-revealing of dietary admission as the reports were taken through food records.

The subsequent investigation estimated the mlx of ADF and exercise which was discovered to be better than fasting or exercise alone as far as lipid levels and changes in weight piece. 64 stout patients were partitioned into four gatherings as referenced. There was a decrease in body weight in the activity just gathering and the mix gatherings. Additionally, the blend bunch had a decrease in LDL, the extent of little high-thickness lipoprotein (HDL) particles (P is equivalent to 0.01), fat mass, and abdomen outline, in any case, the lean mass continued as before. There was likewise an increment in LDL molecule size in ADF just gathering and the mix bunch. The dietary mediation had two periods; a controlled taking care of period (25% of gauge energy necessities) for about a month, and a self-chose taking care of period (food not obligatory) for next about two months. Members in the activity gathering and mix bunch had a moderate force managed practice program three times each week for 12 weeks. At first, they were practicing for 25 minutes which was bit by bit expanded to the term of 40 minutes by week 10. Scarcely any limits of the examination were that it may require over about four months for HDL cholesterol to be modified directed intense exercise. Likewise, practice recurrence and force referenced in the investigation may not be adequate to change the danger pointers of coronary vein infection.

Scientist led an examination to decide if ADF is a decent model of dietary limitation in non-hefty individuals and whether there is any improvement in life span of individuals. They enlisted 16 individuals with eight men and eight ladies who abstained each and every day for 22 days. People lost about 2.5% (P 0.001) of their underlying body weight and 4% of beginning fat mass (P 0.001). Fat oxidation was expanded more than or equivalent to 15 grams in non-hefty subjects, however the yearning didn't diminish on non-fasting days. They suggested that including one little dinner fasting days will make substitute fasting more plausible. Resting metabolic rate and respiratory remainder didn't change essentially from gauge to day 21 and 22 of ADF. There was no huge change in ghrelin and glucose from gauge in substitute fasting subjects while fasting insulin was diminished by 57%. Level of active work fluctuated among the subjects. Seven individuals were stationary, three had moderate movement level and three individuals had exceptionally dynamic life (four to multiple times of activity each week).

The last investigation is a two-year randomized controlled preliminary comprised of 334 patients who were assessed for the impact of intermittent versus on-request admission of extremely low-calorie diet (VLCD) for upkeep of weight in large patients for about four months. The intermittent gathering had VLCD for about fourteen days each third month, while on-request bunch patients had VLCD when the body weight has passed the individual removed level. They had hypo caloric eating regimen during different periods. VLCD-based routine had clinically critical weight reduction following two years. Many danger factors for cardiovascular sickness were improved during the principal year including HDL, LDL, and insulin were improved fundamentally toward the finish of two years of the examination. VLCD had a calorie intake of 450 kilocalories. Ordinary food was gradually introduced during the three-week re-feeding process, during which subjects were given an individualized hypo caloric diet (500 calories per day) for up to two years.

2.4 Discussion

A precise audit of the four examinations talked about showed that intermittent fasting was successful for transient weight reduction. Notwithstanding, there was expanded fluctuation in our included investigations, going from 16 to 334 members with a subsequent period going from three weeks to 104 weeks. Standard attributes of the examination populace were likewise unique as far as weight record which included ordinary weight subjects, overweight and hefty subjects. Method of mediations was likewise extraordinary for every individual investigation.

A methodical survey tracked down that dietary plans had critical weight reduction in intermittent fasting gatherings. In deliberate audit tracked down that intermittent fasting diet was pretty much as powerful as every day limitation of calories both for short and long haul mediations. Most normal issues with persistent calorie limitation diet are that limitation of food constantly is a trigger for higher craving and extra eating. In these circumstances, ADF is a superior arrangement which may be an ideal arrangement so that individuals can eat in their typical manners on non-quick days. This additionally relies upon the kind of the ADF utilized which limits the exhaustion related with ceaseless calorie limitation.

There are restricted information accessible in the writing in regards to the consistency, bearableness, and security of ADF among everyone when utilized as an intercession for weight reduction. It is referenced that insignificant antagonistic impacts, for example, gentle migraines and clogging were knowledgeable about three patients and only one patient was exited the examination as a result of trouble in sticking to the eating routine. A precise survey referenced that there were not many unfriendly impacts identified with the investigation like wooziness and blockage. Hardly any individuals were bad tempered during quick days. Lantz et al. study had a dropout pace of about 65%, likewise there was an absence of low-calorie diet free treatment bunch during the upkeep stage to fill in as a benchmark group.

The dietary program called ceaseless energy limitation (CER) is another successful mean of weight decrease in large and ordinary weight people. It incorporates limitation of day by day calorie admission by 15-60% of pattern energy prerequisites which is commonly extremely difficult to keep up throughout an extensive stretch of time as a result of the need to practice self-guideline and following of the calories. Likewise, CER may make physiologic transformations in the body adjust for calorie limitation which may forestall further weight reduction. Hence, the substitute type of consuming less calories intermittent energy limitation (IER) has been acquiring ubiquity because of its unrivaled viability.

One type of IER is ADF which includes a quick day where members lessen or totally retain any food admission and feed-day in which there is a not indispensable food utilization. The subsequent structure comprises of an entire day fasting remembering total fasting for a couple of days for a week or with 25% of calorie admission in a day with no limitation of nourishment for different days in seven days. The third structure is time limited taking care of where dinners are eaten during explicit occasions in the day, for instance, from 8 am to 5 pm while individuals will stay on fasting for different hours around the same time.

Hardly any biochemical changes related with ADF regarding weight reduction change in mu narcotic receptor qualities, enactment of the dopamine framework, and decrease of D2 dopamine receptor articulation. One of the proposed instruments for the little HDL particles to cause an expansion in coronary illness might be identified with change in the movement of lipases which are related with the development and change of lipoproteins. Expansion in extent of the little LDL particles expands the danger of coronary vein sickness by enlarging oxidization and expansion in porousness of endothelial hindrance.

Benefits of ADF incorporate subject fulfillment without food limitation, tension, and no revealed hyperphagia. Subjects will in general watch what they eat even past the time of calorie limitation as they were utilized to ADF. Individuals who either eat a couple of suppers each day or don't eat anything for significant length of time may show better consistence of ADF diet which may bring about more prominent weight reduction.

Likely detriment of ADF is that it isn't proper for people who are needed to eat dinners at normal stretches, for example, type 1 diabetes, pregnant and breastfeeding ladies, older, people with dietary issues and those needing ordinary food admission to take drugs. Weight reduction for the most part level in a half year, in this manner center around weight upkeep after the underlying time of weight reduction is significant by adherence to low-calorie diet and standard actual work for a more drawn out timeframe.

There were not many examinations with respect to substituting fasting that was led for a brief span of three weeks. It is led an investigation in fat individuals like with a consolidated calorie limitation (decrease in energy consumption by 25%) and directed exercise program (moderate power practice for around an hour for five days in seven days) for twelve weeks. It showed a weight reduction of about 6% from the gauge in the examination bunch. According to blend treatment may cause maintenance of lean mass to the detriment of fat mass during the energy limitation period which thusly assists with keeping up resting metabolic rate in this manner prompted expansions in energy consuming limit and weight reduction. It is referenced that intermittent energy limitation is compelling when contrasted with CER for transient weight reduction with three to five kilograms weight reduction in around 10 weeks.

There are a couple of restrictions related with this orderly audit. Studies that were distributed in different dialects were rejected. Additionally, the area of these investigations were college based settings where members approached top notch food sources, dietician advisors, and guiding from conduct wellbeing individual. Consequently, the outside legitimacy of these examinations was dubious as far as applying it to the country populace who might want to accomplish weight reduction. It was hard to discover for distribution predisposition in our included essential examinations, which may have detailed effective mediations and determination inclination as they would have selected subjects who had high inspiration for adherence to abstain from food. Ultimately, our included examinations were profoundly factor as far as study plan, the creation of the eating routine, measure of energy limitation, the circumstance of fasting period in a day and actual work incorporation as referenced.

Chapter 3. Potential Advantages and Disadvantages of Intermittent Fasting

Intermittent energy limitation (IER) has gotten famous as a methods for weight control among individuals who are overweight and large, and is likewise embraced by typical weight individuals trusting spells of stamped energy limitation will streamline their wellbeing. This audit sums up randomized examinations of intermittent and isoenergetic persistent energy limitation for weight reduction to oversee overweight and stoutness. It additionally sums up the possible advantageous or unfavorable impacts of IER on body structure, fat stores and metabolic impacts from human investigations, including concentrates among typical weight subjects and pertinent creature experimentation. Six little present moment (6 month) concentrates among overweight or stout people show that intermittent energy limitation is equivalent to ceaseless limitation for weight reduction, with one investigation announcing more prominent decreases in muscle versus fat, and two examinations revealing more noteworthy decreases in HOMA insulin obstruction in light of IER, with no conspicuous proof of damage. Studies among typical weight subjects and distinctive creature models feature the possible gainful and unfavorable impacts of intermittent contrasted with ceaseless energy limitation on ectopic and instinctive fat stores, adipocyte size, insulin obstruction, and metabolic adaptability. The more extended term advantages or damages of IER among individuals who are overweight or corpulent, and especially among typical weight subjects, isn't known and is a need for additional examination.

3.1 Introduction
Overabundance energy consumption, weight acquire and ensuing adiposity are reliably connected to disease, handicap and mortality. Randomized preliminaries show that purposeful weight reduction diminishes type 2 diabetes, all-cause mortality and increments psychological and actual capacity. The medical advantages of weight reduction and energy limitation in these human clinical preliminaries are upheld by a hundred years of lab research in rodents, which has set up that energy limitation (ER) forestalls age-related sickness including tumors, cardiovascular infection, diabetes and dementia; impedes maturing related useful decay; and builds life expectancy.

Generally human and creature concentrates on weight reduction have included consistent energy limitation (CER) regulated consistently. All the more as of late, interest has zeroed in on intermittent energy limitation (IER) characterized as times of energy limitation sprinkled with ordinary energy consumption.

IER is of likely interest to oversee stoutness and its metabolic spin-off and furthermore for ordinary weight subjects expecting to advance their wellbeing autonomous of weight reduction for two fundamental reasons: initially, IER just requires the person to zero in on ER for characterized days during the week which is possibly more feasible than the standard methodology of CER which is related with helpless consistence; and, also, numerous useful metabolic impacts accomplished with weight reduction and energy limitation are identified with the energy limitation essentially and are lessened when the individual is not, at this point in pessimistic energy balance. It is thusly conceivable that rehashed spells of checked ER for short spells during the week could give metabolic advantages to post large people past the time of weight reduction who are not, at this point in antagonistic energy balance. IER may likewise give metabolic advantages to typical weight subjects, albeit this requires further examination.

The most contemplated IER approaches are either two back to back long stretches of ER each week ("multi day") or substitute long stretches of ER (ADER), ordinarily with a limitation which is 60%–70% underneath assessed prerequisites, or an absolute quick on substitute days. Confusingly, every one of the three systems have been classified "intermittent fasting" in the writing. In this survey we will utilize the term intermittent energy limitation (IER) to cover these methodologies, "multi day" for two back to back days out of each week, substitute day energy limitation (ADER) when limitation is 60%–70% each and every other day and intermittent fasting (IF) when there is no energy admission on substitute days. It is critical to recognize IF from other IER regimens which permit food on limited days as though may bring out more noteworthy metabolic changes (for instance expanded free unsaturated fats (FFA) and ketones), instigate pressure in people and might be related with hyperphagia during non-confined days.

The increased logical and lay interest in IER among overweight and ordinary weight subjects, demonstrates a need to sum up and assess the viability and metabolic impacts of IER contrasted and CER and evaluate the wellbeing of IER. Ongoing IER audits feature the general scarcity of human information and inferred that IER is similar to CER for weight reduction with little proof of a metabolic benefit. Anyway in many investigations IER and CER were not coordinated for energy admission. Moreover, commentators didn't consider the impacts of IER among typical weight subjects or the significant issue of likely mischief of IER. This account audit will inspect how IER contrasts and CER as far as weight reduction, metabolic changes and security.

3.2 Methods

We incorporate preliminaries of IER with brief times of in any event half energy limitation (7 days) sprinkled with long stretches of ordinary eating (10% energy limitation), however not investigations of Ramadan, limitation for a couple of hours inside the day (time confined taking care of) or concentrates with broadened confined periods, e.g., 2–5 weeks of eating less junk food and not eating fewer carbs which are trying distinctive conduct standards to week by week IER.

To think about adherence and weight reduction accomplishment among IER and CER we incorporate just randomized correlations of IER and CER among free living people where the recommended counts calories had been coordinated for in general energy admission. IER and IF are probably going to effectsly affect metabolic results of interest, e.g., insulin opposition and REE during confined and non–limited stages. Therefore, the metabolic impacts of IF and IER have just been accounted for from considers where creators have expressed that estimations were attempted on limited or non-confined days, which is basic to depict the in general metabolic impacts of the IF and IER regimens.

Intermittent fasting and IER Associated with Greater Weight Control

We distinguished 13 randomized examinations of IER and CER. Seven of the investigations were avoided on the grounds that energy admission was not comparable between the IER and CER gatherings. ADER is the most contemplated IER among people, anyway the majority of these investigations summed up in late surveys have either a no treatment examination bunch or no correlation bunch as were excluded.

We present information on adherence and weight change with IER versus CER for the excess six investigations. These preliminaries tried diverse IER regimens; three tried a multi-day IER one a multi-day IER, one an exchanging example of three to seven days of IER each week and one investigation tried ADER. The majority of the IER regimens prompted smart dieting on the non-confined days. The preliminaries were moderately little with somewhere in the range of 32 and 115 subjects randomized and somewhere in the range of 25 and 88 completers inside the preliminaries. The preliminaries were not fueled to identify contrasts in body weight, and were generally brief length (12–26 weeks). Drop out from the examinations was somewhere in the range of 0% and 40% and essentially practically identical between the IER and CER gatherings, and to past reports inside CER considers. Five of the examinations detailed a goal to get investigation represent these nonconformists.

The entirety of the chose considers show tantamount decreases in body weight among IER and CER. Four of the examinations report identical decreases in muscle to fat ratio; while one detailed a more prominent loss of muscle to fat ratio with two distinctive low carb IER regimens contrasted and CER over a four-month time span. The two IER regimens in this investigation permitted two continuous days out of every seven day stretch of either a low carb, low energy IER (50 grams carb/day) or a less prohibitive low sugar IER which permitted not indispensable protein and not obligatory monounsaturated unsaturated fats. Both had 5 days of a sound Mediterranean sort diet, (45% energy from low glycaemic load carbs, 30% fat; 15% MUFA, 8% polyunsaturated unsaturated fats and 7% soaked unsaturated fats). The IER regimens were contrasted with an isoenergetic 25% CER Mediterranean sort diet. The distinctions in generally starch admission between the eating routine gatherings were unobtrusive (41% and 37% of energy for the two IER slims down contrasted with 47% of energy for CER), which is probably not going to represent contrasts in adherence and decreases in adiposity between the weight control plans.

Adherence to intermittent fasting and IER

Adherence to consume less calories inside preliminaries is famously hard to survey because of missing dietary records and all around archived underreporting among overweight subjects. This in any case, dietary records in four of the investigations gave some data of the relative adherence and by and large energy admission of IER versus CER which was extensively equivalent between the two gatherings.

Two of the investigations of a two-day IER investigated week by week adherence to the ER days and furthermore consumption on mediating non-limited days to survey whether there is any proof of energy remuneration on nowadays. The primary examination utilized a straightforward IER with two continuous confined long periods of 2.73 MJ, from milk, leafy foods. An expectation to treat examination accepting ladies who left the investigation or who didn't finish food records were non-follower detailed that mean (95% CI) 66% (55%–77%) of the potential IER days were finished. The low starch IER tried in the subsequent investigation, permitted a bigger scope of food sources than the recently tried routine and seemed to have a more prominent adherence; mean (95% CI) potential IER days finished for the low sugar, low energy IER and the less prohibitive IER were separately 76% (67%–81%) and 74% (64%–84%).

Neither of the IER tried were related with compensatory hyperphagia on the non-slimming down days. These preliminaries have rather detailed a significant "continue impact" of decreased energy consumption by 20% on non-confined days. Energy consumption on the non-confined days of the IER routine was like the arranged 25% limitation of the CER routine. Food records among the CER bunch in this examination showed that 55% were accomplishing their everyday 25% and a by and large 25% CER. In this manner the more noteworthy loss of fat revealed with the multi day low sugar IER consumes less calories contrasted with CER in the 2013 examination has all the earmarks of being connected to better dietary adherence with IER versus CER, somewhat connected to great adherence to the two limited days every week and the unconstrained limitation of energy admission on non-confined days.

Energy admission was not introduced in the RCT of ADER contrasted with CER, anyway past reports of ADER have also tracked down a little persist impact with a 5% decrease in energy on the non-limited days of the routine. Various examinations were trying joined IER/CER and exercise mediations and revealed exercise to be possible close by both IER and CER counts calories, however there are no detailed associations between diet allotment and levels of action and weight reduction.

Intermittent Fasting and IER helps in Maintaining Weight Loss

Dietary methodologies should show the capacity to keep up weight reduction. Evaluations of fruitful weight reduction upkeep with CER (characterized as 10% weight reduction kept up at a year), change somewhere in the range of 20% and half relying upon the degree of help gave at later time focuses. There are not many information on weight reduction upkeep utilizing IER. One month of a weight support IER (one day of ER and six days of a not obligatory Mediterranean sort diet each week) effectively kept up decreases in weight and of insulin obstruction which had been accomplished with a quarter of a year of a weight reduction IER (two days of ER and five days of a not indispensable Mediterranean sort diet) in the 2013 IER preliminary portrayed previously. In any case, one month is too short a period to make any inferences about the more extended term viability of IER. They had recently revealed that following a half year of counting calories, 58% of the IER bunch contrasted with 85% of CER subjects intended to proceed with the eating routine apportioned at randomization.

Unpublished information from this preliminary show, by a year, 33% of the underlying IER randomization bunch were all the while undertaking a couple of long stretches of IER every week. A goal to treat examination dependent on last perception conveyed forward showed no distinction in the level of ladies in the IER and CER bunches losing 5%–10% of body weight (25% sections 30%) or losing 10% or more at a year.

In synopsis, randomized preliminaries to date have discovered IER to be comparable to CER for weight reduction in six investigations and better than CER for lessening muscle to fat ratio in one examination. All examinations were generally little and in the creator's assessments simply controlled to show total contrasts of 4%–5% between the gatherings. Bigger examinations would be needed to explore if there are more modest contrasts in weight reduction among IER and CER regimens (2%–3% weight reduction contrasts), which would in any case be clinically significant. Studies were primarily directed among ladies and included spurred gatherings of subjects who had addressed adverts, or were selected from a center for ladies at expanded danger of bosom disease. Intercessions have been present moment at 26 weeks, and tried under profoundly regulated conditions with significant degrees of dietetic help and in some cases feast arrangement. Bigger, longer term, true weight reduction preliminaries are needed to educate how IER performs longer term in an assortment of settings in contrast with the standard methodology of CER.

Intermittent Fasting and IER helps in Prevention of Weight Gain in Normal Weight People

There are right now no randomized information to analyze the general viability of IER versus CER to forestall grown-up weight acquire among ordinary weight subjects. Two investigations have tried the metabolic impacts of IER among gatherings of typical and overweight subjects (BMI 20–30 Kg). These examinations have been intended to survey momentary metabolic impacts, chiefly for a little while and included profoundly controlled circumstances in which members were told to expand dietary admission on non–limited days to guarantee they didn't have a general energy shortfall. The examinations report supported appetite with IF, and challenges keeping up every day living exercises during confined days of an ADER routine. This recommends restricted consistence and adequacy of these particular regimens among companions of ordinary and overweight subjects. Notwithstanding, different examples of IER, e.g., one limited day out of each week, might be better endured and warrant study.

3.4 Metabolic Effects of Intermittent Fasting and IER

Decreases in adiposity, explicitly instinctive and ectopic (i.e., hepatic/stomach and intramuscular) fat stores are a restorative objective of ER. Hepatic and instinctive fat stores quickly assemble with checked ER as they are believed to be more delicate to the lipolytic impacts of catecholamine during negative energy balance than subcutaneous fat. Stamped CER (half ER) is identified with fast abatements in hepatic fat in individuals with weight. It is accounted for a 30% decrease in hepatic fat following seven days of a 60%–70% CER in subjects with type 2 diabetes (nine men and two ladies), which standardized hepatic insulin affectability. There are as of now no human information concerning the long haul or ongoing impacts of IER on hepatic, intra-stomach and intramyocellular fatty substance stores. Reports of huge decreases in hepatic fat stores (29%) following two days of ER and carb limitation in people with weight, recommend decreases could happen during the rehashed spells of limitation with IF/IER every week. Such decreases may represent the detailed enhancements in homeostatic model appraisal (HOMA) insulin obstruction, i.e., hepatic insulin opposition with IER portrayed underneath, yet require further investigation.

Interestingly, momentary fasting considers raise the chance of damage with IER among ordinary weight subjects. Times of IER every week will initiate lipolysis and motions in FFAs. The 1–2 days of IF/IER every week will prompt huge transitions in FFA which are commonly three-overlap more prominent than those seen after a typical overnight quick, and will be bigger with IF instead of IER. These motions can prompt skeletal muscle insulin opposition. Single episodes of absolute diets (24–48 hours) in non-large subjects have been related with unassuming expansions in hepatic and intramyocellular fatty substance content which are not seen after the typical 12 hours short-term quick. Explicitly a solitary spell of fasting of between 24–48 hours prompts unassuming expansions in intramyocellular fatty oils (2.4%–3.6%) however not hepatic fat in non-large premenopausal ladies, fundamentally in the second 24 hours' time of fasting, while men have humble expansions in hepatic fat (0.42%–0.74%) inside the initial 24 hours of fasting, yet don't collect intramyocellular fatty oils. The clinical meaning of the humble changes in hepatic fatty substances in men, and intramyocellular fatty oils in ladies in these momentary investigations isn't known. Some however not all investigations have related expanded intramyocellular fatty substances with diminished insulin affectability upon re-taking care of among ladies. Potential systems for expanded hepatic fat with fasting in men incorporate decreased Apo lipoprotein B-100 creation and hepatic lipid send out, as well as debilitated mitochondrial capacity and fat oxidation coming about because of expanded oxidative pressure, with redirection of unsaturated fats for esterification. The impacts of rehashed IER every week on hepatic and intramyocellular fatty substance stores and entire body insulin affectability should be surveyed in longer term considers and furthermore among individuals who are overweight or corpulent.

Adipocyte Size and Adipose Stores

Studies in rodents report blended impacts of IER versus CER on hepatic and instinctive fat stores. One month of substitute long stretches of one or the other fasting or a 75% or 85% energy limitation without a general energy limitation in female subject didn't change weight or aggregate sums of muscle versus fat, yet prompted rearrangement of fat from instinctive (40%) to subcutaneous stores (65%). A comparative examination among male subject didn't track down that substitute long stretches of fasting or ER had consequences for absolute or instinctive fat stores. Nonetheless, in this investigation, substitute days of a half ER and not obligatory taking care of diminished fat cell size in the inguinal (subcutaneous) fat cushions by half and in epididymal (instinctive) fat cushions by 35% [51], regardless of there being no general energy limitation. Checked decreases in fat cell size are thought to diminish hazard of irritation and metabolic illnesses.

Anyway in other creature models rodents and LDL-receptor knockout subject IF regimens decreased energy admission and weight yet expanded instinctive fat, fat cell size and effect insulin affectability contrasted with heavier not indispensable took care of creatures. The variable impacts of IER versus CER on fat stores in various creature models implies extrapolating discoveries from explicit creature models to the human circumstance is dangerous. The unfriendly impacts of IF in these investigations might be since, supposing that creatures embrace a glutting example of eating which thusly can move typical evening brushing to an example of overloading during light hours. This unsettling influence of circadian rhythms may prompt the revealed gathering of stomach and hepatic fat and antagonistic metabolic impacts. The unfriendly impacts of fasting and ER found in these rat contemplates are essential to consider, however may not be an issue for people. As opposed to rat examines, individuals who are overweight or large endeavor IER seem to decrease consumption on the non-confined days and don't show compensatory overloading. The impacts of IER and CER on circadian cadence is significant, anyway this has not been examined.

3.5 Human Studies of Fat Free Mass

Weight reduction and weight upkeep diets ought to diminish muscle to fat ratio stores and, quite far, protect FFM to keep up actual capacity and constrict decreases in resting REE and help to forestall weight acquire. CER is known to lessen FFM notwithstanding muscle to fat ratio. Ordinarily 10%–60% of weight decrease utilizing CER is FFM, contingent upon introductory muscle versus fat, the level of energy limitation, degree of activity and protein consumption. Defenders of IER and IF counts calories guarantee they may protect FFM more than CER from cross investigation examinations of IER and CER mediations which may have permitted our Paleolithic agrarian predecessors to endure spells of food deficiency. Anyway the worry is that spells of extreme limitation with IER and IF (i.e., fasting or admissions of 2.0 MJ/day) could prompt more noteworthy misfortunes of FFM than the unassuming every day energy limitation with CER. There are, be that as it may, not many information to educate this inquiry, as the unobtrusive estimated IER preliminaries attempted are probably not going to be controlled adequately to show distinction in FFM misfortune. Weight reduction preliminaries among individuals who are overweight or large propose misfortunes of FFM with IER and CER are comparable inside the limits of little numbers and are reliant upon the general protein substance of the IER and CER diet as opposed to the example of energy limitation. The primary IER preliminary revealed an identical deficiency of weight as FFM among IER and CER (both 20% of weight reduction) when the two eating regimens gave 0.9 g protein/kg body weight. In like manner the 2013 preliminary announced equivalent misfortunes of FFM (both 30% of weight reduction) with a standard protein IER (1.0 g protein/kg body weight) contrasted with a standard protein CER (1.0 g protein/kg body weight). There was anyway a more noteworthy safeguarding of FFM (20% of weight reduction) with a high protein IER (1.2 g protein/kg weight) contrasted with the standard protein CER (30% with 1.0 g protein/kg body weight (p is equivalent to 0.05). It is accounted for 27% of weight reduction from FFM with IER and CER which both gave 0.7 g protein/kg body weight. Investigations of ADER revealed the extent of weight lost as FFM as low as 10% in ladies with corpulence and as high as 30% among non-large subjects. Ensuing examinations show that activity assists with holding FFM among subjects going through IER and ADER which is very much archived with CER.

One investigation surveyed muscle protein turnover when 14 days of substitute day fasting in typical weight sound men. This examination detailed brought down unthinking objective of rapamycin phosphorylation in muscle which was thought to reflect diminished muscle protein blend and an inability to decrease muscle proteolysis. These progressions could prompt a diminished bulk, accordingly proposing that drawn out substitute day fasting could prompt decreased bulk in ordinary weight subjects.

Resting Energy Expenditure in Human Studies

Resting energy consumption represents 60% to 75% of the complete every day energy prerequisite in an individual, in this way it is significant in deciding in general energy equilibrium and whether an individual is weight stable or acquiring or getting more fit. REE is known to be decreased during CER in relationship with diminished FFM and fat mass, just as to lessen flowing leptin and thyroid chemicals and thoughtful nerve movement. All out energy consumption might be diminished 10% inside about fourteen days of beginning 25% CER.

There are not many information on the impacts of IER on REE. REE could be intensely diminished during the short limited time frames every week, which could standardize during the typical eating days of the week. In any case, an increment in REE of 5% is seen during the primary long stretches of starvation, maybe subsequently to the expanded energy cost of unsaturated fat reusing, glucose stockpiling, gluconeoegenesis, and expanded thoughtful anxious action and catecholamine fixations. Studies to date have surveyed REE after non-confined long periods of IER and have for the most part shown decreases in REE among subjects who are overweight or corpulent and overweight or a typical weight. One exemption is a new preliminary of ADF among 26 subjects with weight, where REE diminished with CER however not IER. Most examinations propose IER brings out similar versatile reaction as CER at any rate on non-confined days. Future investigations ought to evaluate the impacts of IER on REE during limited days to survey the general effect of IER on metabolic rate.

Insulin follows up on skeletal muscle to build glucose take-up and repress protein catabolism, on fat tissue to expand glucose take-up, lipogenesis, lipoprotein lipase and take-up of fatty substances, and on the liver to decrease lipolysis, gluconeogenesis and expands glycogen amalgamation. Heftiness is related with both fringe and hepatic insulin opposition where ordinary or raised insulin levels have a constricted organic reaction in these tissues. Studies in corpulent, overweight and typical weight subjects have evaluated the impacts of IER on entire body, fringe and hepatic insulin affectability utilizing an assortment of strategies, with variable outcomes.

We surveyed HOMA insulin obstruction, a proportion of hepatic insulin affectability, in two RCTS of a two-day IER versus CER among subjects who are overweight or large. As demonstrated over, the principal preliminary looked at IER (two back to back long stretches of 70% ER each week) to an isoenergetic CER (25% ER Mediterranean sort diet seven days of the week) among 105 sound ladies. The IER prompted more noteworthy decreases in HOMA contrasted with CER when estimated on the morning following five ordinary eating days. The mean (95% CI) % change in HOMA more than a half year IER was 24 and CER was 4, (p is equivalent to 0.001). We likewise estimated HOMA on the morning after the two energy confined days, which showed an extra 25% decrease contrasted and CER right now. These distinctions in insulin affectability happened regardless of practically identical decreases in muscle to fat ratio between the gatherings.

The subsequent investigation tried two low carb IER regimens which permitted two successive days out of every seven day stretch of either a low carb, low energy IER (70% ER, 2.7 MJ, 50 g sugar each day) or a less prohibitive low carb IER which permitted not obligatory protein and MUFA (55% ER, 4.18 MJ, 50 g carb each day). These regimens prompted identical decreases in muscle to fat ratio which were both more noteworthy than CER as portrayed previously. Notwithstanding, decreases in serum insulin and HOMA insulin opposition estimated after non-confined days were essentially lower than CER just with the lower energy IER (p is equivalent to 0.02), however not the less prohibitive IER routine (p is equivalent to 0.21). The purposes behind the clear more noteworthy improvement in insulin opposition with more prohibitive IER is autonomous of changes in muscle versus fat and might be explicitly connected to the more stamped energy limitation on confined days (70% stanzas 55%). A new little preliminary among 26 subjects with heftiness detailed fruitful weight reduction with intermittent fasting IF, 8.8 (0.9) % or a 16% CER, 6.2 (0.9) %. Notwithstanding, neither one of the groups experienced changes in insulin obstruction surveyed utilizing an insulin-expanded regularly inspected intravenous glucose resilience test estimated following a non-confined day.

There are not many information of the impacts of IER versus CER on glucose control among overweight and fat people with type 2 diabetes detailed that a multi-day IER more than 12 weeks prompted identical decreases in rate muscle versus fat and in HbA1c contrasted and isoenergetic CER albeit this little examination may have been underpowered to show huge contrasts. Carter detailed comparable decreases in HbA1c in people with

Type 2 diabetes with 12 weeks of IER or CER which had been accomplished with more prominent (but non-critical) decreases in insulin meds inside the IER bunch. It is surveyed the impact of improving a standard 25% CER diet with times of 75% ER (either five days out of each week at regular intervals or one day out of every week for 15 weeks). Typically, extra times of ER expanded weight reduction. The five days of the week intercession brought about the best standardization of HbA1c, autonomous of weight reduction, proposing a potential explicit insulin-sharpening impact of this example of IER added to CER.

Three examinations evaluated the impacts of a little while of IF (exchanging 20–24 h times of a complete quick sprinkled with 24–28 h times of hyperphagia (175%–200% of assessed energy prerequisites). They were intended to guarantee there was no general energy deficiency or weight reduction, and results have shifted between the investigations. It is surveyed the impacts of about fourteen days of IF (an all-out quick for 20 hours from 22.00 and finishing at 18.00 the next day) in eight overweight young fellows. Enhancements in insulin intervened entire body glucose take-up and insulin instigated restraint of fat tissue lipolysis evaluated utilizing an euglycaemic hyperinsulinaemic clasp were seen when estimated following two typical taking care of days, which the creators recommended might be identified with higher adiponectin focuses seen during the 20 hours quick. It is tried an indistinguishable fourteen day intermittent fasting IF intercession in ordinary weight men in a get over plan. Be that as it may IF was not related with changes in fringe glucose take-up or hepatic insulin affectability evaluated with a hyperinsulinaemic clip, or lipid or protein digestion. It is surveyed the impacts of three weeks of IF (substituting 24 hours all out quick and 24 hours not obligatory taking care of) among 16 overweight people. Glucose take-up during a test feast was surveyed at standard following a 12 hours quick and following three weeks of IF on the morning following a fasting day, i.e., following a 36-hours quick. Men had a critical decrease in insulin reaction and improved glucose take-up and insulin affectability, while ladies had disabled glucose take-up and clear skeletal muscle insulin opposition. This perception is probably going to be identified with more noteworthy motions of FFA during this 36-hour quick among fasting ladies, which in all likelihood mirrors an ordinary physiological variation to fasting instead of a reason for concern.

Diminished glucose take-up in skeletal muscle restricts the opposition between skeletal muscle and the focal sensory system and other glucose commit tissues for circling glucose in circumstances with low glucose accessibility, which lessens gluconeogenesis and has protein saving impacts thus has protein saving impacts. The transient investigations of IF illustrated above report blended outcomes on fringe and hepatic insulin affectability and raise the chance of various reactions to IF as per sex. Further investigations are required utilizing strong proportions of insulin affectability.

Studies in other Subjects

Variable impacts of IF regimens on insulin affectability have likewise been accounted for in creature examines. It is tried whether energy limitation with intermittent fasting IF could forestall the improvement of muscle insulin obstruction initiated by a high fat eating regimen. Youthful male rodents were given a high fat eating regimen for about a month and afterward distributed to a proceeded with high fat eating routine (n is equivalent to 12) or an IF with substitute long periods of fasting and a not obligatory high fat eating regimen for about a month and a half. These creatures were contrasted and a gathering who had been taken care of a 36% CER chow diet for the multi week study (n is equivalent to 12). The IF and CER rodents had a diminished weight (IF 27%, CER 14%), and decreased intra-stomach muscle to fat ratio (IF 39%, CER half) contrasted with the high fat eating routine took care of creatures. Whenever neglected to improve insulin invigorated glucose take-up in muscles (estimated following a feed day) regardless of their lower adiposity. Both IF and not indispensable took care of creatures had decreases in muscle GLUT–4 proteins contrasted with CER (30% and 42%). Notwithstanding IF creatures had expanded serum centralizations of adiponectin (92%) and diminished HOMA insulin obstruction (49%) contrasted with the high fat took care of creatures showing improved hepatic insulin affectability with IF. Along these lines, in this creature model, IF favorably affected hepatic, however not muscle insulin opposition contrasted and CER.

The clear more prominent decreases in HOMA insulin obstruction with a multi-day IER contrasted and CER in premenopausal ladies who are overweight or large, and in some pertinent creature models raises the likelihood that IER may improve hepatic insulin affectability. Notwithstanding, IER didn't seem to inspire more prominent upgrades in insulin affectability than CER in three other human comparator preliminaries.

In the event that has been appeared to effect fringe and hepatic insulin invigorated take-up of glucose in non-corpulent subjects. The wellbeing ramifications of rehashed transient expansions in FFA and expansions in fringe insulin opposition with IF and IER every week are not known and need further examination. This might be especially significant for bunches which experience the biggest transitions of FFA, i.e., ordinary weight people and ladies.

3.7 Intermittent Fasting and Metabolic Flexibility

Times of energy limitation or delayed exercise switch liver, skeletal muscle and heart tissues to fat oxidation, and the catabolism of amino acids, while the post prandial state favors glucose take-up and oxidation. The corresponding guideline of fat and glucose oxidation is controlled deliberately by insulin and glucagon, and because of changes in cell levels of metabolites like unsaturated fats, pyruvate, citrate and malonyl CoA which direct mitochondrial catalysts. Energy digestion is viewed as ideal when the body can promptly switch between oxidizing glucose or fat because of supplement accessibility and physiological pressure. This is considered to keep up metabolic wellbeing and the ideal cell working. The switch in energy digestion is known as metabolic adaptability. Metabolic rigidity is seen in overloaded people who don't handily switch among fat and glucose oxidation. There is concurrent oxidation of fat, glucose and amino acids all of which increment oxidative pressure, diacylglycerols, ceramides, and acylation of mitochondrial proteins, which thusly brings about bothers of mitochondrial work. Metabolic resoluteness is believed to be the underlying driver of insulin opposition.

Particular times of ER sprinkled with ordinary energy admission every week might be much the same as agrarian ways of life and may advance support of metabolic adaptability contrasted with standard day by day slims down, particularly since IER contains longer times of ER than our typical overnight quick. A new report in rodents of ADF upholds this idea. Male rodents were exposed to 48 days of IF (eight rehashed patterns of three days of fasting and three days re-taking care of) or an isoenergetic 20% CER. The IF subject appeared guideline of qualities for both lipid stockpiling and fat oxidation reflecting great metabolic adaptability with expanded fat oxidation during fasting days and lipogenesis on non-confined long stretches of IF. These progressions were not initiated with an isoenergetic 20% CER.

In people, a half year of a 25% CER has been appeared to improve metabolic adaptability, as proven by expanded change in fasting-to-postprandial groupings of acyl carnitine (significant for move of unsaturated fats into the mitochondrion before oxidation). There are presently no information of the impacts of IER on metabolic adaptability in people.

Is IER Safe like Intermittent Fasting?

There are hypothetical worries that IER could advance flighty eating designs, gorging, and low disposition. A new orderly audit of 15 clinical preliminaries presumed that checked CER (60%) decreased gorging conduct among overweight or large people with pre-treatment pigging out jumble, and didn't seem to trigger voraciously consuming food in those without past voraciously consuming food problem. It is accounted for decreases in despondency and voraciously consuming food and improved self-perception insight following two months of following ADER. Interestingly, a month of IER (four sequential days of a 70% ER and three days of not obligatory eating) among nine typical weight young ladies, named intemperate eaters, brought about expanded sensations of craving, more regrettable temperament, elevated crabbiness, challenges concentrating, expanded weariness, eating-related musings, dread of loss of control and over eating during non-confined days [80]. We have announced equivalent decreases in profile of mind-set state scores for pressure, despondency, outrage, exhaustion and disarray, an expansion in life and a general decrease in absolute temperament unsettling influence with a multi-day IER and CER. Hence existing information show IER can improve eating practices and temperament among subjects with overweight and stoutness, yet may have the potential for hurt among ordinary weight people with unreasonable eating styles.

Another regular concern is whether the spells of checked energy limitation with IER could annoy the hypothalamic-pituitary-gonadal hub in ladies and adjust the recurrence and length of monthly cycles. Such impacts are probably going to be identified with the beginning load of the individual, generally energy balance and the quantity of continuous limited days with IER. The 2011 IER concentrate among fat and overweight ladies announced a more extended normal period length in ladies following IER for a half year (two successive long stretches of 70% ER each week) contrasted with 25% CER bunch. An examination among typical weight, stationary, ordinary cycling ladies tracked down that three sequential days of an all-out quick during the mid-follicular stage influenced luteinizing chemical elements, yet were lacking to irritate follicle advancement, or period length. The impact of IER on the regenerative pivot among large, overweight and typical weight subjects requires further examination, particularly regimens which incorporate longer times of energy limitation.

IER doesn't seem to restrict a people's capacity to work out. A multi week consolidated ADER and exercise preliminary among subjects with stoutness announced equivalent participation to a managed practice program (40 min of 75% max pulse on three days out of every week) on both limited and non-confined long periods of ADER. Also it is accounted for a tantamount expansion in every day normal advance include in the IER and CER gatherings and detailed practically identical and great adherence to a moderate power strolling program (five 20–50 min meetings of energetic strolling 60%–70% max pulse each week) among calorie counters undertaking IER and CER.

Most of contemplated IER regimens have suggested good dieting and not devouring non-limited days. Devouring non-limited long periods of IER effects wellbeing, notwithstanding weight reduction. For instance, a high fat ADER (45% fat) created comparable weight reduction to a low fat ADER. Nonetheless, regardless of weight reduction in this examination, the high fat ADER bunch had diminished brachial course stream interceded expansion which could expand hazard of atherosclerosis and hypertension.

In this way, restricted information to date recommend that IER isn't related with cluttered or voraciously consuming food, irritation of the hypothalamic-pituitary-gonadal hub, and doesn't restrict the capacity to practice among in people who are overweight or fat. Anyway the security longer term and among typical weight people isn't known.

Optimal IER Regimen

The ideal span, recurrence and seriousness of ER needs to find some kind of harmony of being reachable, while likewise conveying guessed gainful metabolic impacts. There are various possible changes of IER and IF which could be considered. IER is probably going to be desirable over IF regimens among people, as it is probably going to have more prominent consistence and lower pressure and cortisol reactions. IER regimens may have to give some energy and protein consumption on limited days (i.e., 2.5 MJ and 50 grams protein) to keep up nitrogen equilibrium and FFM, which doesn't appear to be accomplished with spells of complete fasting. IER summons more modest variances in FFAs and ketones than IF. The last is connected to momentary debilitated glucose resilience during the resumption of ordinary taking care of. The more drawn out term ramifications of momentary disabilities in glucose resistance with rehashed IF every week isn't known.

The circumstance of energy admission during the limited long periods of IER doesn't give off an impression of being significant for consistence and weight announced equivalent decreases in weight with a 75% ADER with it is possible that one supper at lunch or supper or three little dinners for the duration of the day.

3.8 Discussion

This survey features an absence of excellent information to educate adherence and advantages or damages regarding IER versus CER. Examination discoveries and holes in the proof contrasting IER with CER for weight control and metabolic wellbeing are summed up. The couple of randomized examinations of IER versus CER among overweight and hefty subjects report identical weight reduction, with one preliminary of a multi-day low sugar IER revealing more noteworthy decreases in muscle to fat ratio contrasted with CER. These examinations were not fueled to recognize a distinction in deficiency of weight or fat, accordingly study finding are intriguing yet not decisive of no contrast among IER and CER. No examinations to date have tried whether IER can forestall weight acquire among typical weight subjects, anyway IER regimens dependent on substitute long stretches of complete fasting or stamped energy limitation (70% limitation) have not been all around endured among ordinary and overweight populaces (BMI 20–30 kg).

This survey features various holes in information on the impacts of IER stanzas CER on ectopic and instinctive fat stores, adipocyte size, FFM, insulin obstruction, REE and metabolic adaptability, especially among ordinary weight subjects. Without these information, we have drawn on discoveries of momentary investigations and featured some possible helpful or unfriendly impacts. The variable and in some cases unfavorable impacts of IER on fat stores and digestion in some subject revealed in this survey are a worry. In any case, this may relate to a limited extent to shifts in night and day eating designs and circadian beat, which may not mean the human circumstance.

Future IER research requires two sorts of randomized correlation preliminaries. Right off the bat, longer term RCTs of IER and CER (a half year) to show whether IER is reasonable long haul and has long haul benefits or yet unseen hurtful impacts on weight, body creation, and metabolic wellbeing contrasted with CER. Besides, point by point metabolic evidence of standard examinations in controlled conditions to evaluate the impacts of IER and coordinated isoenergetic CER on FFM, hepatic and intramuscular fat stores, insulin affectability and metabolic adaptability utilizing powerful system, for example, DXA, MRI and insulin clips. These investigations need to survey the metabolic impacts of IER during limited and feed periods of the eating regimen to completely portray its natural impacts among individuals of any weight.

All around archived contrasts in metabolic reactions to times of fasting and stamped energy limitation between pre-menopausal ladies (i.e., expanded ketones and free unsaturated fats) contrasted with men and post-menopausal ladies propose conceivable diverse metabolic reactions, and maybe better resistance to IER inside specific populaces. Future IER studies ought to incorporate guys, more established subjects, and people with dreary stoutness or type 2 diabetes, just as would be expected weight subjects. There is additionally a need to investigate ideal examples of limitation, e.g., two days of the week, substitute days, five days out of each month [86] or different changes and the best method of limitation on the confined and interceding days (e.g., low carb, low protein).

The fame of IER inside the overall population combined with the holes in the proof we have distinguished demonstrate that IER merits further thorough investigation. We don't know decisively whether long haul IER is a safe powerful technique for weight control for subjects who are overweight or stout or whether IER may give medical advantages to individuals of any weight autonomous of weight reduction. Great exploration looking at long haul results of IER and CER are needed to determine any obvious advantages or hindering impacts which IER may have for controlling weight and improving metabolic wellbeing in the populace.

Chapter 4. Intermittent Fasting Effectiveness to Reduce Body Mass Index

The impacts of an intermittent fasting diet (IFD) in everybody are as yet questionable. In this investigation, we planned to efficiently assess the viability of an IFD to lessen weight file and glucose digestion in everyone without diabetes mellitus. Data sets were looked to distinguish randomized controlled preliminaries and controlled clinical preliminaries that contrasted an IFD and a customary eating regimen or a nonstop calorie limitation diet. The adequacy of an IFD was assessed by the weighted mean distinction (WMD) for a few factors related with glucometabolic boundaries including weight file (BMI) and fasting glucose. The pooled mean contrasts of results were determined utilizing an intermittent impacts model. From 2814 examinations distinguished through a writing search, we at last chosen 12 articles (545 members). Contrasted and a control diet, an IFD was related with a huge decrease in BMI fasting glucose level and homeostatic model evaluation of insulin opposition. Fat mass would in general diminish in the IFD bunch with a critical expansion in adiponectin, an abatement in leptin levels. An IFD may give a critical metabolic advantage by improving glycemic control, insulin obstruction, and adipokine focus with a decrease of BMI in grown-ups.

4.1 Introduction

Calorie limitation (CR) is known not exclusively to diminish body weight yet additionally to improve different cardiovascular danger factors. Delayed CR has been appeared to lessen fat mass with critical weight reduction. An improvement of insulin obstruction was additionally recognized after CR. Components of CR-interceded improvement of glucose digestion are not completely clarified, however potentially include critical changes in insulin affectability of skeletal muscle, alongside the decrease of fat mass.

INTERMITTENT FASTING & BMI

By and by, there are numerous challenges in supporting day by day CR. As an elective eating regimen intercession to CR, weight control through intermittent fasting (IF) has been proposed. An assortment of diets have been utilized to consider the impacts of IF, including substitute day fasting (ADF, burning-through no calories on fasting days), substitute day adjusted fasting (ADMF, devouring under 25% of benchmark energy needs on fasting days), time-limited fasting (TRF, confining food admission to explicit time-frames of the day), and occasional fasting (PF, fasting simply one to multi day out of every week). Notwithstanding the impact on weight reduction, numerous investigations have shown that through IF we can expect an incredible impact on progress of glucose digestion by bringing down insulin opposition, improvement of foundational fiery sicknesses assurance against neurodegeneration, and even extension of the life expectancy.

In a new report, an IF diet (IFD) improved insulin affectability in any event, when the provided calories were equivalent to those of the benchmark group, without critical change in body weight. This shows that IF, itself, can be valuable to glucose digestion autonomous of body weight changes, notwithstanding, in spite of different outcomes, in some controlled, randomized hybrid preliminaries, IF didn't improve glucose and lipid digestion. Moreover, there were additionally clashing outcomes in the impact of weight decrease. Albeit a few investigations revealed critical weight decrease in an IFD bunch, a few different preliminaries didn't report a clinically significant weight decrease.

As seen from the changed and conflicting discoveries of past examinations, numerous obstacles dependent on the qualities of the eating routine intercession study, like non-normalized dietary control of the patient, low consistence, and the quantity of members because of the trouble of leading an investigation covering a whole period, and the trouble of setting the benchmark group, make it hard to recognize the advantageous impacts of an IFD. Moreover, a few past meta-examination concentrates on the glucometabolic impact of an IFD have likewise shown clashing outcomes, which is significant for building up diet proposals for everybody incorporating the populace with weight or pre diabetes. Accordingly, this examination planned to explore the viability of IF on weight reduction and glucose digestion by dissecting the impact size of past investigations among everyone without diabetes mellitus (DM).

4.2 Eligibility Criteria

The incorporation rules of the writing were as per the following: concentrates on everyone without persistent sicknesses that could influence glucose digestion including diabetes mellitus (patients, P); those that considered an IFD (intercession, I); those that thought about the benchmark groups, standard eating regimen (RD) or consistent CR diet control without fasting (12 hours) (correlation, C); and those that depicted fasting glucose, homeostatic model evaluation of insulin opposition (HOMA-IR), absolute body weight, weight file (BMI), fit mass, fat mass, leptin, and adiponectin (result, O) as indicated by the exploration question (PICO). Just controlled preliminaries of administered diet programs were qualified. Studies were restricted to intercessions which were a base a month in length. Likewise, just investigations that introduced the mean and standard deviation of the outcomes were chosen.

We barred examinations on patients with diabetes mellitus, ongoing liver illness, constant renal sickness, and studies on pregnancy (P); those that elaborate a blend with explicit supplement limitation diet mediation (I); those that contrasted and an alternate kind of IFD (C); and those with results other than the boundary of glucose digestion, like mental boundary (O). The writing was freely chosen by two scientists and instances of intermittentities were settled by means of an exhaustive conversation. Regarding the likelihood that a few articles could be missed by the above search terms, we further looked through the audit papers of comparable points to check whether there were any papers relating to a similar information extraction.

Fasting glucose, HOMA, BMI, fat mass, slender mass, leptin, adiponectin, and complete body weight were utilized as factors for the impact of an IFD and were determined utilizing the mean, standard deviation, number of members, just as pattern and last qualities. The substance of the writing were inspected in detail, and the sorts of IFD and control diet were coded and introduced. On the off chance that there was a mathematical outcome because of the distinctive benchmark group in the substance of one record, the information were separated by classifications for the benchmark group and mistakes coming about because of the duplication of similar reports were enhanced utilizing measurable procedures.

Analysis of Stats

To enhance the precise audit, a meta-investigation was performed. It was utilized to incorporate the impact sizes of the 12 chose records. The weighted mean contrast (WMD) between the standard and last estimations of fasting glucose, HOMA-IR, BMI, fat mass, fit mass, leptin, adiponectin, and complete body weight as indicated by the intercession were considered as the impact size, and the opposite fluctuation strategy was utilized in light of the fact that the qualities were ceaseless factors. The arbitrary impacts model was picked due to the variety and heterogeneity of the intercession. Heterogeneity was assessed utilizing the I2 measurement across the investigations. I2 esteems were deciphered as follows: 0% to 40%, no significant heterogeneity; 30% to 60%, moderate; half to 90%, generous; and 75% to 100%, impressive heterogeneity. The heterogeneity of pooled impacts between subgroups was determined utilizing measurement. A pipe plot technique was utilized to test potential distribution inclination.

4.3 Results

A sum of 2814 examinations were chosen by the hunt technique for our investigation. Subsequent to taking out 1216 copy records, the titles and modified works of 1598 investigations were looked into, and 1097 papers that had no significance with the first survey as indicated by the PICO were avoided. Among 501 examinations chose by investigating the titles and modified works, 12 examinations were at last remembered for this examination. The absolute number of members was 545 (261 in the mediation bunch and 284 in the benchmark group; 210 or 38.5% men and 335 or 61.5% ladies).

Impact of Intermittent Fasting on BMI

An aggregate of eight investigations provided details regarding the impacts of an IFD on BMI. Seven examinations evaluated diet intercession just, and one of the investigations surveyed diet mediation with work out, which was similarly surveyed in the benchmark group. No distinction was seen between the two gatherings for BMI at benchmark. After the eating regimen mediation, BMI was fundamentally lower in the IFD bunch by 0.75 kg. The IFD was additionally connected with a pattern towards lessening body weight. A sum of 10 examinations covered the impacts of an IFD on body weight. All subtleties of the progressions in body weight were introduced in kilograms (kg). No distinction in body weight at standard was seen between the two gatherings. The heaviness of the members was lower in the IFD bunch by 1.94 kg, without factual importance.

Impact of intermittent fasting (IF) versus a non-fasting control on weight record (changes from benchmark) in grown-ups without constant metabolic infection. The squares show the investigation explicit result gauges, and the size of the squares compares to the examination's weight in the meta-investigation. Level lines signify the scope of the 95% certainty span. The jewels show pooled gauges. Loads are from arbitrary impacts investigation.

A sum of eight investigations gave an account of the viability of an IFD to diminish fasting glucose levels. Six examinations evaluated an IFD in particular, and two different investigations surveyed an IFD with work out. No distinction was seen between the two gatherings in fasting glucose at benchmark. After intercession, a critical lessening in fasting glucose level was affirmed. An IFD was likewise connected with brought down HOMA. A sum of six examinations wrote about the adequacy of an IFD to decrease HOMA-IR levels. The HOMA levels of the members were lower in the IFD bunch by 0.54 after diet mediation.

Not show huge contrasts between the two gatherings, both in the standard and after diet intercession. In spite of the fact that without measurable importance, an IFD was related with a pattern towards diminishing fat mass. The fat mass was higher in the IFD bunch at pattern, in any case, it was lower after mediation. Despite the fact that there was no huge change in fat mass after an IFD, an IFD was related with an expansion in adiponectin level and a reduction in leptin level; without the distinction in the pattern.

4.4 Discussion

The best quality level administration of heftiness or overweight is 20% to 30% CR alongside a far reaching way of life alteration, notwithstanding, bounce back weight acquire is a genuine issue of weight decrease the executives in clinical circumstances. As of late, an IFD has been acquiring ubiquity as an elective technique for accomplishing and keeping up weight decrease. Considering the disparity of IFD viability on glucose digestion and the absence of proof in meta-investigations, we led a methodical pursuit and chose 12 examinations. Based on this meta-investigation, we affirmed an improvement of fasting blood glucose and insulin opposition through IFD as contrasted and a non-fasting control bunch. This is by all accounts identified with an abatement in the BMI and a leptin level decrease, just as an increment in adiponectin level. Lean mass was generally preserved in the IFD bunch, nonetheless, no huge weight decrease was recognized. In past investigations, the general weight decrease of both an IFD and a day by day CR (by 15% to 60% of the typical caloric admission consistently) were comparable between two gatherings. In this investigation, the examination of complete body weight incorporated an extra paper with more serious level of consistent CR diet as a benchmark group, which clarifies why there was a genuinely extraordinary error between absolute body weight and BMI in this investigation.

Regarding IFD adequacy on glucose digestion, numerous difficulties remain. In some past investigations, the impact of IFD on blood glucose was not huge, and there were various discoveries as per the qualities of members. A 3% to 6% decline in fasting glucose was seen in patients with pre diabetes, though no huge impact on fasting glucose focus was seen in solid people. In this examination, we incorporated all investigations of members with or without pre diabetes, in light of the fact that the meaning of pre diabetes was frequently indistinct in past examinations. Accordingly, we discovered an improvement in blood glucose and insulin obstruction in everybody with the incorporation of some corpulent with pre diabetes populace gatherings. Insulin obstruction is related with DM advancement. Thusly, IFD may be more valuable to patients with high insulin opposition who are probably going to advance to DM.

The advantageous impacts of an IFD remembering impacts for glucose digestion are regularly respected to be driven by decreases in body weight or potentially muscle to fat ratio. Past IFD contemplates that embraced ADMF or ADF diet intercession with a moderately serious level of CR brought about clinically significant decreases in body weight, while a generally little (5.0 kg) weight decrease was accomplished in IFD examines receiving a TRF diet with little level of CR. Furthermore, no critical weight reduction was seen in investigations that changed the fasting time while keeping up the all-out calorie admission. Along these lines, the fundamental pathophysiologic system of weight reduction through an IFD is probably going to be a decrease in the complete calories burned-through. In this investigation, no critical weight reduction was seen in the IFD bunch when contrasted with the non-fasting control bunch. The fundamental clarification for this outcome may be the blended attributes of the benchmark group including both consistent CR and RD gatherings. All things considered, a propensity toward weight decrease was seen in the IFD bunch and a critical decline was seen in the examination with BMI.

Roughly one-fourth to 33% of weight decrease is known to be of lean tissue during constant CR, be that as it may, lean mass has been saved in many past investigations under an IF diet mediation. Also, in this examination, lean mass didn't show a critical contrast when the eating routine intercession. Adjusting boosting loss of muscle versus fat and limiting loss of slender mass is one of the significant pathophysiologic ways to deal with keeping up actual capacity and decreasing insulin opposition. The preservation of lean mass may have added to the expansion of HOMA decrease.

Albeit fat mass decrease during an IFD was not genuinely huge, after mediation, a critical expansion in adiponectin level and a diminishing in leptin level were noticed. Leptin and adiponectin are fat tissue inferred chemicals and are related with glucose digestion. Lower leptin focuses are by and large joined by a decrease of fat mass. Adiponectin levels are adversely connected with insulin opposition, fat mass, and focal fat conveyance, and dependent on this investigation, we propose that an IFD is by all accounts related with an improved dispersion of focal fat.

Thinking about the benefits of an IFD and its component of various outcomes when contrasted with consistent CR, consideration has been given to the significance of the fasting time term in past investigations. Following 12 hours of fasting, lipolysis begins in fat tissue and afterward moves digestion from fat stockpiling and lipid union to activation of fat as a type of unsaturated fat determined ketones. This can be required to lessen fat mass and improve insulin obstruction. With comparative calorie admission decreases during persistent CR, this distinction in fasting time influences the mass and circulation of fat tissue, at long last having an effect in glucose digestion, just as adipokine level changes. Furthermore, as a normal benefit of IFD in contrast with consistent CR, an IFD can be supported with higher consistence and could have a more huge impact on fat mass decrease and insulin obstruction all through the fasting period.

The relationship of circadian cadence with an IFD is a significant issue. In a new report, expanded danger of cardiovascular infection was accounted for in a populace without or with just a basic breakfast. Skipping breakfast is related with an increment in the arrival of stress chemicals. Also, there was an examination showing that essentially improved weight reduction and improved insulin obstruction were seen in a gathering that burned-through more calories in the first part of the day and less in the evening, in conditions with the comparative calorie limitation. The kind of intercessions in the examinations remembered for this investigation were very assorted, and there was an impediment to additional examination. Randomized controlled preliminaries under refined conditions could be useful to explain the relationship with circadian musicality.

This examination had some different limits. In the first place, just investigations that introduced the mean and standard deviation of the benchmark and end-product with a benchmark group were chosen. Hence, the quantity of members remembered for the examination was little. Second, we just incorporated everyone without ongoing metabolic infection, and along these lines we were unable to decide through this investigation whether an IFD is compelling in patients with persistent metabolic sickness, for example, diabetes mellitus. The intercession bunch included different sorts of IF, and the level of calorie limitation shifted likewise. The non-fasting control bunches likewise went from RD to persistent CR. Notwithstanding this variety, the subgroup examination was restricted because of the deficient number of studies. Concerning the mathematical highlights of members, including identity, a few examinations showed heterogeneous attributes and others didn't gave adequate data, and thusly we were unable to lead further investigation. Third, since the chose concentrates all had intercessions of present moment (four to 24 weeks) span, it is restricted to anticipate long haul impacts of IFD.

In certain regards, these restrictions may fill in as qualities. This examination was led to break down just refined investigations with a benchmark group. The members of this examination address everybody with a wide scope of BMI, and accordingly affirm the IF adequacy on all inclusive community without persistent metabolic illness. Through this investigation, we found that IF improves glucose digestion through lipolysis by affirming the distinction in BMI, HOMA-IR, leptin level, and adiponectin focus among the members. Through the consequences of this investigation, we can anticipate an improvement of fat dispersion during an IFD, in any case, further examinations are needed to explain this advantage of IFD.

Taking everything into account, IF altogether improves glycemic control and insulin obstruction with a decrease in BMI, a reduction in leptin level, and an increment in adiponectin fixation in everybody without persistent metabolic illness.

4.5 Intermittent Fasting and Meal Timing

Stoutness stays a significant general wellbeing concern and intermittent fasting is a famous procedure for weight reduction, which may introduce free medical advantages. Notwithstanding, the quantity of diet books exhorting how fasting can be consolidated into our day by day lives is a few significant degrees more noteworthy than the quantity of preliminaries analyzing whether fasting ought to be supported by any means. This survey will consider the condition of current arrangement with respect to different types of intermittent fasting (for example 5:2, time-confined taking care of and substitute day fasting). The viability of these transiently characterized approaches shows up extensively comparable to that of standard day by day energy limitation, albeit a significant number of these models of intermittent fasting don't include took care of abstained cycles each and every other 24 h rest wake cycle as well as license some restricted energy admission outside of recommended taking care of times. Appropriately, the intercession time frame in this manner may not consistently substitute, may not traverse all or even the greater part of some random day, and may not include outright fasting. This is significant in light of the fact that possibly beneficial physiological instruments may possibly be started if a post-absorptive state is supported by continuous fasting for a more drawn out length than applied in numerous preliminaries. In reality, promising consequences for fat mass and insulin affectability have been accounted for when fasting span is regularly reached out past sixteen sequential hours. Further advancement will require such models to be tried with proper controls to disengage whether any conceivable wellbeing impacts of intermittent fasting are essentially owing to routinely extended post-absorptive periods, or basically to the net negative energy balance by implication evoked by any type of dietary limitation.

Intermittent fasting is a wide term that includes an assortment of projects that control the circumstance of eating events by using transient diets to improve body creation and generally speaking wellbeing. This survey inspects examines led on intermittent fasting projects to decide whether they are compelling at improving body structure and clinical wellbeing markers related with infection. Intermittent fasting conventions can be assembled into substitute day fasting, entire day fasting, and time-limited taking care of. Substitute day fasting preliminaries of 3 to 12 weeks in length give off an impression of being viable at lessening body weight (3%-7%), muscle to fat ratio (3-5.5 kg), complete cholesterol (10%-21%), and fatty oils (14%-42%) in ordinary weight, overweight, and corpulent people. Entire day fasting preliminaries enduring 12 to 24 weeks likewise lessen body weight (3%-9%) and muscle versus fat, and well improve blood lipids (5%-20% decrease in complete cholesterol and 17%-half decrease in fatty oils). Examination on time-confined taking care of is restricted, and clear ends can't be made as of now. Future examinations ought to analyze long haul impacts of intermittent fasting and the likely synergistic impacts of joining intermittent fasting with work out.

Diets using intermittent fasting (IF) as an essential strategy to control body creation have as of late filled in prominence, be that as it may, dietary works on including fasting have likewise been followed for quite a long time for strict reasons (i.e., Ramadan). Notwithstanding the explanations behind participating in IF, the effects on slender weight (LBM) might be unfavorable. Past research has shown that opposition preparing advances LBM gathering, nonetheless, regardless of whether this actually happens during IF is indistinct. Thusly, the goal of this audit is to deliberately dissect human examinations researching the impacts of varieties of IF joined with obstruction preparing on changes in LBM in beforehand inactive or prepared (non-world class) people. Changes in body weight and fat mass, and convention adherence were surveyed as an auxiliary goal. This survey followed the favored announcing things for orderly audits and meta-examinations data sets were looked for articles researching IF, joined with opposition preparing that detailed proportions of body organization. Eight investigations met the qualification rules. LBM was by and large kept up, while one investigation announced a huge expansion in LBM. Muscle versus fat mass or rate was essentially decreased in five of eight investigations. Results propose that IF matched with obstruction preparing by and large looks after LBM, and can likewise advance fat misfortune. Future examination ought to inspect longer-term impacts of different types of IF joined with opposition preparing contrasted with customary types of energy limitation.

In the course of the last 10 to 15 years, intermittent fasting has arisen as a whimsical way to deal with decrease body weight and improve metabolic wellbeing past straightforward calorie limitation. In this survey, we sum up discoveries identified with Ramadan and Sunnah fasting. We at that point examine the part of caloric limitation as an intercession for weight control, yet significantly, as a methodology for sound maturing and life span. At long last, we audit the four most basic intermittent fasting (IF) procedures used to date for weight the board and to improve cardio metabolic wellbeing. Weight reduction is regular after IF yet doesn't have all the earmarks of being not the same as day by day caloric limitation when thought about straightforwardly. On the off chance that may likewise give extra cardio metabolic advantage, like insulin sharpening, that is autonomous from weight reduction. While no particular fasting routine stands apart as unrivaled as of now, there is in reality heterogeneity in reactions to these extraordinary IF eats less carbs. This recommends that one dietary routine may not be undeniably appropriate for each person. Future examinations ought to think about methodologies for fitting dietary solutions, including IF, in view of cutting edge phenol composing and genotyping before diet inception.

The point was to determinate if the intermittent fasting improves weight reduction or muscle gains in people more youthful than 60 years of age. Various data sets were looked up to May 2020 for concentrates in English, utilizing terms and text words relating intermittent fasting, weight reduction and muscle gains. The convention was enrolled in PROSPERO. Study quality was evaluated utilizing NICE strategy. An aggregate of 10 unique articles were assessed. Eight papers gathered information through randomized controlled preliminaries and two from cross-sectional investigation. Intermittent fasting could be useful in opposition prepared subjects or in overweight people to improve body arrangement by diminishing fat mass and at any rate keep up bulk; decline in GLP-1 levels and; improving wellbeing related biomarkers such glucose and insulin levels. Be that as it may, future examinations are required to all the more likely explain the impact of intermittent fasting on body arrangement.

Different intermittent fasting (IF) dietary plans have acquired notoriety among hefty people as of late as a methods for accomplishing weight reduction. In any case, contemplates assessing the impact of IF regimens in individuals with metabolic condition, pre diabetes and type 2 diabetes (T2D) are restricted. The point of the current survey was to momentarily clarify the biochemical and physiological instruments hidden the constructive outcomes of IF, particularly the impact of the proposed 'metabolic switch' on digestion. Then, we analyzed the adequacy and wellbeing of IF regimens in people with metabolic condition, pre diabetes and T2D. To accomplish this, we played out a search utilizing mixes of different IF terms, remembering preliminaries for which members met the extra rules for metabolic disorder, pre diabetes or T2D. We discovered four investigations in people with metabolic disorder, one examination in individuals with pre diabetes, and eight investigations in individuals with T2D assessing the impacts of various IF regimens. The restricted accessible proof, with little example sizes and short preliminary spans, recommends that IF regimens have a comparative adequacy contrasted and calorie-limitation abstains from food for weight reduction and improvement in glycemic factors. When all is said in done, most IF regimens are powerful and safe. Be that as it may, there is an expanded danger of hypoglycemia in patients with T2D who are treated with insulin or sulphonylureas. Besides, long haul adherence to these regimens seems questionable. There is a requirement for huge controlled randomized preliminaries to assess the adequacy of IF regimens, particularly in people with metabolic disorder and pre diabetes. Whenever demonstrated to be reasonable and solid for delayed periods, IF could offer a promising way to deal with improving wellbeing at the populace level, and would bring about various general medical advantages.

That eating design comes in a few assortments. A few plans call for limiting eating to a 6-to 12-hour window each day. Others call for eating ordinarily a couple of days seven days, at that point profoundly limiting calories for 2 or 3 days. The two methodologies have been appeared to help, with concentrates in the domains of weight reduction and metabolic wellbeing showing specific guarantee. One late 12-week investigation of overweight ladies in their 40s tracked down that the individuals who ate just 500 calories, 3 days out of each week, and didn't limit calories the other 4 days, lost the same amount of weight as the individuals who slice calories to an exacting 1,200 to 1,500 day by day. Furthermore, in a 6-month preliminary including 100 ladies, half were allotted to a 5:2 intermittent fasting plan (fasting 2 days and eating what they needed the other 5) and the other half to an eating regimen where they cut every day calories by a quarter. The two gatherings lost a similar measure of weight, yet those in the 5:2 gathering lost more gut fat.

Indeed, even without weight reduction, fasting can help fight off diabetes and heart issues, examines recommend. In one late University of Alabama study, pre diabetic men who restricted their eating from 9 a.m. to 3 p.m. for 5 weeks, while as yet eating enough to keep up their weight, saw improved insulin affectability and pulse. What's more, investigations of strict gatherings have shown that fasting as little as a day a month for the long haul can influence heart wellbeing and life span. 2,000 patients for a very long time and tracked down that the standard fasters were 45% more averse to pass on during the investigation time frame and 71% less inclined to have cardiovascular breakdown. The individuals who had abstained the greater part of their day to day routines additionally by and large experienced longer.

Maybe the most captivating yet least investigated advantage lies in cerebrum wellbeing. Researchers have known for quite a long time that ketones, which are delivered when the body is famished of sugars and can infiltrate the cerebrum can be a powerful fuel hotspot for synapses and quiet "thunderstorms" or seizures in the individuals who have a sort of epilepsy. Fasting can likewise animate creation of the nervousness suppressing synapse GABA. Also, creature examines have shown that intermittent fasting can forestall synapse demise, fight off Alzheimer's-like manifestations, and lift the capacity to learn and recall.

Conclusion

The efficient audit of the previously mentioned four investigations tracked down that intermittent fasting was powerful for transient weight reduction among ordinary weight, overweight and corpulent individuals. Randomized controlled preliminaries with long haul follow-up period are expected to follow the adherence to count calories and long haul upkeep of weight reduction without recapturing the shed pounds. Future examinations ought to likewise incorporate explicit subgroups of the populace, for example, people with cardiovascular danger factors and type 2 diabetes mellitus as these patient populace advantage more from weight reduction which may change the sickness cycle. In outline, corpulence and overweight is a global wellbeing emergency, and intercessions, for example, ADF are expected to assist individuals with accomplishing weight reduction.

Lightning Source UK Ltd.
Milton Keynes UK
UKHW020651280521
384539UK00010B/624